Table of Contents

Introduction

This book is part of a series of books, which are here to help you find natural solutions for many of the issues you encounter every day, be it a beauty concern, a household malfunction or just curiosity to learn more about how to use the gifts of Nature directly, in the purest condition possible.

The central idea, around which the topics of this book revolve is the incredibly multiple ways in which a natural product, as simple as one lemon, can be used. I was always amazed at the power of nature every time it came to natural remedies and homemade products, and this was the main reason why I started working on this book.

In the first chapter "Lemon Recipes for Beauty" I gathered the simplest recipes and tips which will help you avoid many of the mainstream beauty products, so you can save time, money, and stay away from artificial colors and preservatives.

The second chapter, entitled "Home Remedies and First Aid Using Lemon" will help in an emergency situation and teach you how to cure minor trauma and common diseases at home and without medication.

The third chapter "Lemon for Healthier Life" does not deal with emergencies, but is in no way less important. It will provide you with tips on how to naturally improve and maintain your precious health through a very simple lemony daily routine.

Finally, the fourth and last chapter of this book, "How to Use

Lemon at Home", is aimed to assist you with the house chores and to avoid chemical cleaning agents. It will provide you with precious tips and hacks, and save you time and money for much more pleasant activities.

I hope you will find this book useful, as I wrote it especially for those people who want to care for themselves and the people they love.

Chapter 1
Lemon Recipes for Beauty

How far can one lemon go to make you more beautiful? You'll be surprised! In this chapter, I will give you numerous ways by which lemons can improve your physical appearance by resolving skin problems and other dilemmas!

If you're ready, let's get it on!

Knee and Elbow Bleacher

If your knees and elbows appear dark, it is because in these areas, the skin is thicker and drier, and it is prone to hyperpigmentation. Lemon is known for its exfoliating, softening and bleaching effects. With this simple tip, your knees and elbows will gradually become lighter, giving your whole skin a more even tone.

Ingredients:

One fresh lemon cut in half

Directions:

Rub your knees and elbows with half of the lemon once or twice a day. If the lemon is still juicy after the first application, you can reuse it, but keep it stored in the fridge, wrapped in a plastic sheet or bag.

Be careful not to rub lemon into wounded skin.

Treat Blackheads

Lemons also have antioxidant and antibiotic effects, which means they can be used for blackhead treatment. If your skin is very oily, prone to acne and outbreaks, lemon juice is what will help treat and prevent spots, blackheads and oiliness.

Ingredients:

Freshly squeezed lemon juice.

Directions:

Wash your face as usual. Apply lemon juice on clean and dry skin, using a piece of cotton or a cotton pad. Let the juice dry for a couple of minutes, then rinse with water and follow your usual treatment or moisturizing routine. Spots and blackheads will begin to disappear after a couple of days.

Note: If your skin is very dry or very sensitive, use lemon juice on damp skin to avoid irritation and moisturize properly after rinsing.

No More Problematic Skin

Another product for problematic skin, which you can make at home, is this lemon juice and tea tree essential oil skin toner. What's more, this can also be used with cotton pads as a cleansing wipe. It is ideal for oily and combination skin types, which are acne and blackhead prone. Lemon prevents the bacteria to spread, deodorizes the skin and closes large pores. Tea tree essential oil soothes and revitalizes the skin.

Ingredients:

3 drops of freshly squeezed lemon juice

2 drops of tea tree essential oil

2 tablespoons of distilled water

Directions:

Mix the three ingredients in a small cup, dip a piece of cotton or a cotton pad in the mixture and apply on your face instead of your regular toner; it can also be utilized as a cleansing to remove impurities from the pores.

Lemon for Teeth Whitening

Lemon juice combined with baking soda can do miracles to your teeth.

It is very common that over time, even the naturally white teeth lose their sparkle. Coffee, tea, soft drinks and juices are to blame for the gradual tooth pigmentation. Try this simple recipe, with which you can whiten your teeth easily without having them covered in chemicals or paying a fortune to a dentist.

Ingredients:

3 tablespoons of baking soda

2 tablespoons of freshly squeezed lemon juice

Directions:

Mix the baking soda and the lemon juice and apply the paste to your teeth using a clean Q-tip. Let it work for 5 minutes. Then scrub your teeth and gum with a toothbrush and rinse thoroughly.

Bonus effect: not only will your teeth become whiter, but your gums will also become stronger, as it improves blood circulation. You're welcome!

Lemon for Brighter Skin

One of the most famous benefits of using lemon on skin is their brightening and lightening effect. Freckles, dark pigmented patches, unsuccessful fake tan and age spots on face and hands can be significantly lightened, or even completely removed with lemon. Try this home recipe for brighter and softer skin.

Ingredients:

¼ cup white sugar

3 tablespoons of freshly squeezed lemon juice

1 tablespoon of grated lemon zest

Directions:

Mix sugar and lemon zest together and add the juice. Apply the paste to the area you want to lighten. Massage gently and allow it to dry on the skin for 5-10 minutes, then rinse with warm water. Apply it daily, and after the 3rd-4th application your skin will become noticeably brighter.

Note: Lemon juice makes the skin more sensitive to UV rays, so don't forget to wear a sunscreen before going out in the sun after therapy.

Say Goodbye to Chapped Lips

Chapped lips are unwelcome for many reasons: the feeling of dryness both for you and whoever comes in contact with them is almost unforgivable! Plus, the lipstick looks cracked and messy, spoiling even the neatest makeup. Dehydration is the number one cause for chapped lips, so first of all check your daily water intake. However, sometimes even when your body is properly hydrated, your lips could still look chapped. This means that the problem lies on the surface! Below is a recipe which will help remove dead skin cells from your lips, so they will quickly become soft again.

Ingredients:

A tiny amount of freshly squeezed lemon juice

Directions:

Dip your finger into the lemon juice and spread it on your lips before bedtime. Rinse in the morning.

Note: Do not use lemon juice on lips that have cracks. Let them heal first.

Perfect DIY Manicure

It's not only the skin and hair which could benefit from lemons; if your nails have yellowed, are dry and tired from gel manicures, are brittle or splitting, there is a simple way to treat them at home.

Ingredients:

Freshly squeezed lemon juice
Olive or any other oil
White vinegar
Water

Directions:

Mix equal parts of lemon juice and oil in a manicure bowl and soak your nails for about 10 minutes. Rinse with warm water and wipe them dry. Prepare a solution of white vinegar with water in equal parts and brush your nails with it.

Lemon has bleaching and softening properties; oil nourishes and moisturizes the nails and the skin around them. The white vinegar polishes the nail's surface.
Follow this routine once a week and keep your nails in great shape!

Skip the Dye with Lemon

Want to naturally lighten your hair or make some dye-free highlights? All you need is lemons and a sunny day!

Ingredients:

¾ cup of freshly squeezed lemon juice
¼ cup water

Directions:

Mix juice and water together. Put the mixture in a spray bottle and spritz your hair thoroughly before going out in the sun. The time of exposure depends on how lighter you want your hair to become and also on how strong the sunlight is. It generally ranges between 30 minutes and one hour.

After the exposure wash your hair as usual and use a moisturizing conditioner or hair mask, as lemon increases your hair's sensitivity to sunlight and they might become more dry and fragile.

Do not expose your hair to sunlight for too long if it is already damaged. In this case it might also be better if you changed the lemon-water proportion to 1:1.

After 2-3 days of sunlight working with lemon on your hair you will notice some light, beautiful and all-natural highlights!

Simple Dandruff Treatment

An itchy, flaky scalp is obviously neither pleasant nor beautiful. Before spending money on doubtfully effective shampoos and treatments, why not try this DIY dandruff therapy with lemon? Lemon juice contains Vitamin C and citric acid, which help the skin regenerate, and this is exactly what is needed to get rid of the white flakes.

Ingredients:

3 tablespoons of freshly squeezed lemon juice
2 cups of water

Directions:

Before washing your hair, mix the juice with water. Before using your regular shampoo, apply the mixture on wet scalp and massage gently for 2 minutes. Then rinse and follow your usual washing routine. Repeat the treatment every second day until dandruff is gone.

It usually takes up to 3 weeks.

Treatment for Super Acneic Skin

We already know that lemon treatment clears up blackheads and prevents the formation of new ones because of the salicylic acid it contains. But there is another, even stronger recipe to treat severe acne. Acneic skin needs extreme doses of salicylic acid to clear up and look healthier, so we will now combine lemon with aspirin, which is the acid we need here.

Ingredients:

1 tablespoon of freshly squeezed lemon juice
10 uncoated aspirin pills

Directions:

Crush the aspirin pills into powder, add the lemon juice and mix into a smooth paste. Wash your face as usual, pat to dry and apply the mask either on the whole face or only on the acneic areas. Let it dry for 10 minutes. You may experience some tingling, but don't worry: it is the salicylic acid working inside your pores. Rinse well and follow your regular moisturizing routine. You will notice the difference immediately!

Facial Exfoliator

If your skin looks dull and is rough to touch, it is certainly time for some gentle exfoliation. Exfoliants and face scrubs available on the market usually contain chemicals and hard particles. These products may seem more effective, but in fact they damage the skin's surface, making it thinner and helpless against the bacteria. Scrubbing the face too hard also provokes quicker keratin formation, which makes the skin rougher and is exactly what we are fighting against here. The following is a tip to exfoliate safely at home, with all-natural ingredients.

Ingredients:

½ cup of raw oats
approx. ¼ cup freshly squeezed lemon juice

Directions:

Pulse the oats in a blender until they become a fine powder, and then slowly add the lemon juice. Put the thick paste on clean skin and let dry for about 10 minutes. Rinse well and moisturize as usual.

Lemon Rinse for Shiny Hair

Your hair may become dull due to a prolonged use of styling products, which cannot be easily removed with regular shampoos. Small particles of hair sprays, gels and foams gather on the surface of the scalp and hair, causing itching, dandruff and dullness.
To make your hair shiny again, all you have to do is to follow this simple procedure.

Ingredients:

2 tablespoons of baking soda
1 cup of lemon juice
2 cups of water

Directions:

Prepare a solution of water and lemon juice. Wash your hair with your regular shampoo. After rinsing, massage your wet scalp with the baking soda for 2 minutes. It will remove the styling products from the skin. Rinse again and pour the lemon juice – water solution on your hair. Let it dry for 2 minutes and rinse thoroughly. Your hair will become shiny again!

Chapter 2
Home Remedies and First Aid Using Lemon

Home Remedies and First aid using natural ingredients seem to be out of the question now that the market can offer "quick fixes". The thing is, these fixes could be dangerous to your health and the health of your family.

Now, let's try to revive the good 'ol ways of curing minor health issues!

Relieve Cough and Get Better Soon

When you are down with a sickness, a productive cough is actually a good thing. During this period the lungs produce more mucus, which destroys the bacteria and removes them from the body with coughing. To assist this natural process and get better faster you should drink plenty of fluids. Tea is a classic. The right tea though is the one that will not only keep you warm and hydrated, but will also relieve the sore throat. Here it is!

Ingredients:

1 teaspoon chamomile tea (any tea would work, but chamomile is the best)
2 teaspoons honey
2 teaspoons fresh lemon juice

Directions:

Brew the chamomile in a large cup of water and wait until it is not very hot. Then add honey and lemon. Drink one cup every 2 hours.

Soothe a Sore Throat

A sore throat is one of the worst cold symptoms for me. Where the pastilles won't work, the lemons come to the rescue!

Ingredients:

¼ cup freshly squeezed lemon juice
½ teaspoon salt

Directions:

Put the ingredients in a cup, fill it with warm (not hot!!!) water and stir to dissolve the salt. Gargle every 1-2 hours. Do not swallow!

Reduce the Fever Naturally

For very high fevers, medication and doctor's advice are a must. For the less extreme cases, though, there is a natural way to help the chills and reduce the fever.

Ingredients:

1 small lemon
2 tablespoons of honey

Directions:

Squeeze the lemon's juice in a cup, add the honey, fill the cup with warm water and stir. Drink the whole solution at once every 2 hours. It will help reduce the fever while keeping you warm.

Cure Corns and Calluses

Corns and calluses are painful and don't easily disappear on their own. There are ways, though, to naturally cure them with lemon.

Ingredients:

1 small slice of lemon
or
lemon essential oil

Directions:

Take the lemon slice and apply it to the corn/callus and fasten it with a band aid. Leave it overnight and repeat for as many times as necessary.

You can also use lemon essential oil instead of a lemon slice. Apply a little oil on the corn/callus with a Q-tip and leave until it is completely absorbed. Be careful not to use undiluted oil on soft skin around the callus, as it can cause burns.

Minor Cuts and Wounds

Until recently, it was considered a common sense that wounds should be cleaned either with hydrogen peroxide or alcohol. Latest evidence shows that the former can cause clots and the latter can burn the skin, actually delaying the healing process. Try a better and safer way to disinfect minor skin trauma.

Ingredients:

lemon juice

Directions:

First, pour clean water on the cut and pat with something clean to dry. Pour lemon juice on the wound to disinfect and stop the bleeding.

Relieve the Wasp Stings

It is significant to distinguish wasp stings from bee stings, because these two require exactly opposite treatments. While the bee sting venom is acidic and it is better neutralized with an alkaline substance, such as baking soda, wasp venom is alkaline, as well as other insect bites, and can be relieved with acid. And here come the lemons!

Ingredients:

Fresh lemon juice

Directions:

Apply a little lemon juice on the sting with a cotton pad or a Q-tip. Let dry and repeat until it feels better.

Canker Sore Treatment

There are many factors which can lead to canker sores formation: from stress, dietary habits and hormonal shifts to severe disease. But no matter the cause, these small unpleasant wounds better heal as soon as possible. Lemon has antibiotic properties and chamomile soothes the mucous membrane.

Ingredients:

1 tablespoon dried chamomile
¼ cup freshly squeezed lemon juice

Directions:

Brew the chamomile in ½ cup hot water and let it cool so it is just warm. A hot infusion is bad for the sores. Add the lemon juice in the chamomile and stir. Gargle with this solution 2-3 times a day until the sores are healed.

Soothe Poison Ivy Rash

If you are among the unlucky ones who are sensitive to the poison ivy oil or to other poisonous plants and have already developed the rash, a simple thing can be done to soothe the itching and help accelerate the healing process.

Ingredients:

Fresh lemon juice

Directions:

Soak a cotton pad in lemon juice and pat on the rash. It may sting a little because of the acid which disinfects the skin.

DIY Motion Sickness Medication

Motion sickness, also known as the Inner Ear Disturbance, can spoil all the fun of traveling. The symptoms of travel sickness appear when the brain receives mixed signals during travel: either when the eyes cannot see the movement the body feels or when the body cannot feel the movement the eyes see. There is no way to alter the brain's functions, but there is something you can do about the symptoms. Next time you are about to take a boat or go out on a road trip, remember of lemons.

Ingredients:

A slice of lemon

Directions:

Suck on the lemon slice to prevent nausea and dizziness or to calm down your already upset stomach.

Aid Your Digestion

Lemon also helps to unblock the digestive system. Constipation is not a minor issue. Chronic costiveness is potentially dangerous, as over time it can transform into very serious diseases including colon cancer. It is thus significant to catch the condition early, or even better – to prevent it. This lemon juice solution is a great supplement to a healthy diet rich in fibers and serves both the treatment and prevention of constipation.

Ingredients:

1/5 cup freshly squeezed lemon juice

Direction:

Fill a cup with warm water and add the lemon juice. Drink once a day to aid digestion. You can also add a teaspoon of honey for better taste.

Remove the Warts

Warts are caused by some very common viruses that settle inside the skin through scratches or wounds. They are really persistent and have the tendency to reappear just when you thought they're finally gone. One home remedy that could help to get rid of warts is the lemon juice.

Ingredients:

Freshly squeezed lemon juice

Directions:

Leave a drop of lemon juice on the wart to dry. Do this daily. The acid will gradually destroy the wart tissues and help the skin heal underneath.

Jellyfish Sting Treatment

Don't let unpleasant things like jellyfish stings spoil your vacation on the beach. To relieve the pain, itching and minimize the rash, just ask for a piece of lemon from the beach bar!

Ingredients:

A piece of fresh lemon

Directions:

Remove any pieces of jellyfish from your skin by gently scraping them off with a credit card or any other card. Rinse the stung area with sea water and squeeze the lemon on it.
If you are at home or in your hotel room, squeeze the lemon juice in a glass and add equal amount of water. Soak a piece of cotton in the solution and put it on the rash.

Chapter 3
Lemon for Healthier Life

Do you need to strengthen your immune system? Or do you have some problems with digestion? If so, lemons can help you! In this chapter, I'll teach you how to maximize the potential of lemons when it comes to building a healthier lifestyle.

A Healthy Drink for Healthy Digestion

Diarrhea, constipation, bloating, heartburn, indigestion, liver problems, kidney disease and many other digestive system problems can be prevented with the use of lemon. Natural acids and vitamins found in lemons assist an easier and healthier digestion. They also improve bowel movement, help the body to get rid of toxins and strengthen the immune system. To get all these digestive benefits, all you have to do is follow this simple routine.

Ingredients:

100 ml freshly squeezed lemon juice

Directions:

Put the lemon juice in a cup and add warm water until it is full. Stir and drink this solution once a day. You can sometimes use slightly warm herbal infusions instead of water. It is this simple!

Lemons for Weight Loss

Dieting is not easy at all, especially on the first week when your body strives with the new regimen and all you can think of is food. It is not that your life is really endangered without the regular amount of food, but your whole body seems to react like this is the end! Pectin fiber, which is very much present in lemons, is the solution. Sour yellow fruits are here to fight the feeling of hunger and help you lose weight without suffering.

Ingredients:

100 ml freshly squeezed lemon juice
2 teaspoons honey

Directions:

Mix the lemon juice and honey in a cup and add warm water. Drink this solution to eliminate the cravings. This drink will also give you energy and it is naturally sweet!

Lemon for Radiant Skin

If you want your skin to be healthier and appear younger at any age, you should give it proper food. Your skin loves Vitamin C and citric acid, which restore the age signs and prevent the appearance of wrinkles and age spots. A balanced diet and exercise can do miracles to your skin, especially if combined with this simple and natural drinking supplement with lemon.

Ingredients:

100 ml freshly squeezed lemon juice

Directions:

Pour the lemon juice in a cup, add warm water and drink daily. If you don't like the sourness, add a teaspoon or two honey so it tastes better. You will notice the benefits within a month.

Keep the Infections Away

Are you sick of getting sick? Boost your immune system and help your body fight infections. Lemon water fills your body with Vitamin C, which helps improve resistance to viruses, and also increases iron absorption. It is better to start early, before you catch the flu: preferably in October. But even if you are already down with an illness, this lemon drink will help you get better soon.

Ingredients:

100 ml freshly squeezed lemon juice

Directions:

Add 150 ml warm water in the cup with the lemon juice, stir and drink once a day for prevention, or every 2 hours with honey and ginger – to get better quickly.

Bad Breath Treatment

Bad breath (also called halitosis) is one of the top embarrassing things you certainly want to treat. The worst thing about having bad breath is that you might be unaware of it, because usually even the closest people are too embarrassed to tell you about this.

The causes of halitosis are many; the most common are: dry mouth, smoking, insufficient oral hygiene, certain foods or medical conditions. In all cases except for a disease, it is possible to eliminate or completely treat halitosis with lemon, as it has great antibacterial and deodorizing properties.

Ingredients:

100 ml freshly squeezed lemon juice
2 teaspoons honey

Directions:

Combine the lemon juice and honey in a cup and fill it with warm water. Stir to dissolve and drink twice a day: before going to bed and after your breakfast. It will neutralize the bacteria in your mouth and hydrate you, giving the ultimate solution to the bad breath problem.

pH Balance for Health

Maintaining the pH levels in your body is important, because extreme acidity is often responsible for increased inflammatory processes, particularly in the soft tissues. Joint pain, kidney stones, bone disease could happen due to excessive acidity, which is also called acidosis. Prevention is always better than treatment, and lemons are here to do the job. Lemon juice is rich in citric and ascorbic acids, which are great alkalizing supplements. All you have to do is to prepare the following.

Ingredients:

Fresh lemon juice

Directions:

Pour some lemon juice in a glass of water and drink this solution every morning on an empty stomach. Maintaining your pH levels is as simple as that!

Level Up Your Energy

Are you feeling tired all the time? You think that you need more energy to live a fuller life, but don't know where to start? I suggest starting with simple, but effective things, like this tasty fruity-lemony DIY energy drink. High in carbohydrates and electrolytes it will instantly fill you with energy! Plus, you can have as much as you want, as it is 100% natural and healthy.

Ingredients:

Juice of ½ lemon
¼ cup fresh fruit juice (whichever is your favorite)
1.5 tablespoons of honey
A pinch of salt

Directions:

Mix the two juices in a glass, add honey and salt and stir until everything is properly blended. Fill the rest of the glass with water, stir again and it's ready! Enjoy every day for full batteries.

Prevent Respiratory Infections

Upper Respiratory Tract Infection -or simply: sore throat, nasal congestion and cough- must be the most "popular" illness in the winter. The annoying symptoms of the infection interfere both with productivity in the workplace and the ability to just relax and sleep, which makes it even worse. How can we boost our immune system and keep the germs away? With Vitamin C, citric and ascorbic acids from lemon, plus the antiviral properties of honey and cinnamon. This beverage is also warming and tastes great; perfect for the cold winter days!

Ingredients:

50 ml freshly squeezed lemon juice
2 tablespoons honey
½ teaspoon cinnamon powder

Directions:

Put the three ingredients in a cup and mix. Add hot water (not very hot!) and stir until the honey is fully dissolved. Enjoy every day to stay warm and prevent colds.

Fix the High Blood Pressure

If your blood pressure is high, you might want to prepare this natural homemade infusion, which consists of peppermint and lemon. Peppermint tea, when consumed regularly, could be helpful in lowering the blood pressure, while lemon juice cleans and hydrates the lymphatic system. Lemon also helps you stay calm and sleep better, which is a very significant part of the treatment.

Ingredients:

1 teaspoon peppermint leaves (fresh or dried)
50 ml lemon juice

Directions:

Brew the peppermint leaves in ¾ cup hot water and let cool. Then add the lemon juice and stir. Drink this infusion once a day to help your body normalize the blood pressure naturally.

Maintain Urinary Tract Healthy

To avoid urinary tract infections (UTIs) and keep the urinary organs healthy it is essential that you drink the right amount of the right fluids every day. Clean water is indisputably vital for our body, but note that in large amounts it can wash a significant percentage of electrolytes away, causing quite opposite effects. One of the fluids which are super beneficial for the health of the urinary system consists of lemon and ginger. The acids of the lemon and the anti-inflammatory properties of ginger make a great match in keeping away the UTIs.

Ingredients:

1 very small piece of ginger (approximately 5 mm thick)
2 tablespoons of freshly squeezed lemon juice

Directions:

Slice the ginger into thin rounds and boil it for 7-10 minutes in a glass of water. Strain the tea and let cool. Add the lemon juice and drink once a day. You can also add a teaspoon of honey for better taste.

Lemon Benefits for Mind and Soul

The use of essential oils is evident in every page of the human history. To this day scientists are still exploring the unimaginable variety of properties of these "magical potions". Citrus essential oil, in particular, is known for its positive impact on the mood and the alertness of the brain. Try inhaling the lemon essential oil scent for a minute and notice your state of mind alter to a more positive and relaxed one. Feeling dizzy? Dampen a handkerchief with lemon essential oil and slowly inhale the scent for a few minutes. Need better concentration at work? Use an air freshener that smells of citrus.
And for better sleep prepare this essential oil mixture.

Ingredients:

1 small drop of the essential oils of lemon, chamomile and valerian (one drop from each)
1 teaspoon of chamomile tea

Directions:

Prepare a chamomile herbal infusion and put the essential oil drops in the cup. Drink before bedtime.

Note: Pets are much more sensitive to essential oils than humans, so be careful when using the oils around your four legged pals.

Lemon Oil for Beautiful Legs

Spider veins and varicose might not be fatal, but they sometimes really add age to your otherwise beautiful legs. There are plenty of surgical methods which promise the best aesthetic results, but are they as safe as they seem? And who would really want to undergo such a procedure to hide some minor flaws? It is always better to try something natural first, so I would suggest this homemade balm with lemon essential oil.

Ingredients:

2 drops of lemon essential oil
½ cup almond oil (avocado, jojoba or another similar oil will also do)

Directions:

Drip the lemon oil into the almond oil and stir. Apply daily on the areas where the small veins are visible and massage softly until the mixture is completely absorbed by the skin.

Chapter 4
How to Use Lemon at Home

Be it cleaning or deodorizing, lemons can help you at home! All you have to do is follow the recipes listed below!

Clean the Microwave

Every single food that you cook or heat in the microwave is leaving its mark. Over time stains and smells gather inside and can become quite unpleasant to clean. And sometimes even after cleaning, the microwave retains the smells of different foods.

Lemon water neutralizes the smells and also makes the cleaning process faster and easier. This is the tip for simpler cleaning.

Ingredients:

¼ cup lemon juice

Directions:

Take a wide shallow plate and fill it with water. Add the lemon juice and put the plate in the microwave. Boil the water on the highest wattage for 10 minutes. Then clean the microwave with a sponge and soap as usual and rinse.

Bonus feature: lemon water also helps you to get rid of the soap remainders completely after cleaning the oven or the fridge.

Sanitize the Cutting Boards

Cutting boards must be the best place for hidden pathogens. Although the boards might look perfectly clean, in most cases they are not. Food remainders stay deep inside the scratches of the chopping boards and decompose, contaminating whatever comes in contact with them. Gross, huh? But there are solutions to the problem!
First of all, prefer plastic to wooden chopping boards. Secondly, use each board for only one type of food: one for meat, one for veggies etc. And last, use this cleaning and deodorizing tip to eliminate the possibilities of contamination.

Ingredients:

Juice of one lemon (for one chopping board)

Directions:

After cleaning the board as usual, pour the lemon juice on the scratched side, leave for 10 minutes and wash again. Lemon will remove the smells and prevent bacteria from "being fruitful and multiplying".

Hide the Unpleasant Smells

It is impossible to keep the garbage disposal perfectly clean and smelling like heaven at all times, because… well, it's a garbage disposal! If you forgot or simply did not have time to make it perfectly clean, at least make it smell better.

Ingredients:

As many used lemons as you have
or
A few drops of lemon essential oil

Directions:

Put the used lemons or some lemon essential oil drops in the garbage to instantly hide the indiscreet smells. And that's it!

Remove Stains from Chinaware

You may have noticed that tea and coffee leave dark stains on the chinaware. These stains don't easily go away, and sometimes persist even after a session or two in the dishwasher. Surprisingly, this happens not because of the tea color or the material of the cups, but due to the water hardness. If the water in your area is rich in calcium, it floats on boiled water as chalk particles and sticks to the sides of the cup. And because these chalk particles take the color from the tea, the stains are dark. With this scrub these stains will vanish immediately!

Ingredients:

½ cup lemon juice
1 cup salt

Directions:

Mix the lemon juice and the salt into a thick paste and rub your cups. Then rinse thoroughly.

Homemade Lemon Flavoring

Various lemon flavorings are available on the market. They may be based on natural lemons, but the chemical preservatives are hard to be omitted when it comes to any food industry. Make a natural DIY lemon extract to flavor water, cakes, drinks or sauces, with only a few ingredients and a little patience.

Ingredients:

2 small lemons (only the skin/zest – no pith)
1.5 teaspoon sugar
¾ cup vodka (40% alcohol)

Directions:

Zest the lemons and put the zest in a dark glass jar or bottle. Add the sugar and the alcohol and stir. Close the bottle with a cap, so no oxygen gets inside and leave it in a cool, dry and dark place. Shake it every day for a month and a half. It is best to wait as long as you can; preferably 3 months. When you decide to use it, strain the mixture first.

Polish for Wooden Surfaces

Wooden furniture requires special maintenance. Chemical polishing agents found on the market don't usually smell good and are quite costly. To hide the tiny scratches and smoothen the surface of wooden furniture naturally, use this simple trick with lemon.

Ingredients:

¼ cup freshly squeezed lemon juice
½ cup olive oil (or any other oil you have in your kitchen)

Directions:

Mix the ingredients in a bowl and polish the wooden surfaces with a cloth or a paper towel to shine.

Lemon Air Freshener Spray

As the writers C. Classen, D. Howes and A. Synnot state in their amazing book *The Cultural History of Smell*, in today's society smells are not really welcome. More and more people prefer the non-smelling environment, as it is associated with sterile cleanliness and high social status. For those romantics who miss the "good old days" which smelled of fruits and flowers, here is a recipe for a homemade spray to create a special aromatic aura.

Ingredients:

2 teaspoons of freshly squeezed lemon juice
2 teaspoons of baking soda
4 drops of lemon essential oil (or any other essential oil)
½ liter hot water

Directions:

Combine the lemon juice, the baking soda and the essential oil in a spray bottle, add the water and shake well until the soda is properly dissolved. Spray as an air freshener. You can also use this solution in potpourri. Smells great!

Clean the Kitchenware

Kitchen utensils in general, and copper pots in particular, tend to discolor and lose their luster over time. Spots, discoloration, burned oil, calcium deposits, all the signs of constant use are quickly becoming visible even on new kitchenware. A safe and cheap way to clean and deodorize pots and utensils is to use lemon.

Ingredients:

1 lemon
a small bowl with salt

Directions:

Cut the lemon in half and press the cut side into the bowl with salt, so as plenty of it sticks to the lemon. Then rub the kitchenware with the salty lemon half, dipping it in salt from time to time, so it retains its scrubbing properties. Let the mix on the utensils for 5 minutes and rinse with warm water. You can also use a cloth dipped in lemon juice to renew clean kitchenware.

Insect Repellent with Lemon

Mainstream insect repellents, which you can find in supermarkets, might be dangerous, as they come in direct contact with bare skin and are absorbed into the body, bringing unnecessary chemicals to our life. They also cause rashes and allergies. In other words, it is better to avoid them. There are plenty of homemade insect repellents based on essential oils and natural ingredients. Here is one of my favorites.

Ingredients:

100 ml freshly squeezed lemon juice
4 tablespoons lemon extract (you can make it at home)
10 drops lavender oil
1.5 cup distilled water

Directions:

In a spray bottle pour the lemon juice, add the lemon extract and the lavender essential oil drops. Fill the bottle with distilled water. Shake well before every use.

Note: Do not use this spray on animals, as they are much more sensitive to the essential oils than us humans, and might develop allergies or breathing problems.

No More Scratches

Big ones or small ones, scratches are inevitable on surfaces of wooden or painted furniture, and plastic or metallic household appliances. Very small scratches can disappear simply by polishing the area with the homemade polishing liquid you will find below. Deep scratches need to be filled first, and then polished.

Ingredients:

½ cup freshly squeezed lemon juice
½ cup any plant oil (I prefer coconut, as it smells great)

Directions:

Mix the lemon juice and the oil in a bowl. Use a hand mixer, as the oil tends to remain on the surface. Dip a soft cloth or a paper towel in the mixture and thoroughly rub the scratches. Do not use excessive amounts of oil-lemon mixture; you don't want the surfaces to become sticky and gather dust.

Clean and Maintain Antique Ivory

Antique ivory jewelry and piano keys get yellowish when exposed to direct sunlight. You need to be careful with cleaning, as although ivory is basically a tooth, it isn't nearly as hard as human teeth. Ivory lacks the enamel, which is hard as diamond. Prepare this mild cleansing to whiten and polish antique ivory. And please do not buy new ivory. No need to kill even more elephants!

Ingredients:

½ cup of freshly squeezed lemon juice
½ cup water

Directions:

Mix the lemon juice with the water in a cup or a bowl. Take a soft absorbent fabric and slightly dampen it with the lemon-water solution. Rub the ivory surface gently until it becomes white again. For hard stains, sprinkle a little fine salt and rub very gently to avoid scratches.

Renew Hardened Paintbrushes

Do not throw the godforsaken hardened paintbrushes away! You can revive them with the power of lemon juice in just a few easy steps. Just make sure the brushes can resist boiling water temperatures, because it is going to be hot, and we don't need victims here.

Ingredients:

½ liter lemon juice

Directions:

Pour the lemon juice into an old kitchen pot and put the hardened brushes in the juice in such way that only the hair of the brush is completely covered in juice. Boil the juice together with the brushes for 15 minutes. Repeat if needed.

Remove Paint from Glass

Painting doors and windows is not an easy job, and it becomes even more unpleasant because of the paint stains on glass that haunt every painter, no matter how well the glass was protected. The good thing is that there is a way apart from scratching the glass or using special chemical paint diluters to remove the dried paint stains. Here is a natural paint remover you can find in your kitchen.

Ingredients:

½ cup of freshly squeezed lemon juice

Directions:

Pour the lemon juice in a small pot and warm it until it starts to boil. Carefully dip a small piece of cotton in the hot juice. It is best to use tweezers with a plastic handle. Place the juicy cotton piece on the paint stain and pat it so it sticks to the glass. Remove the cotton after 20 minutes and wipe the paint off.

Lemon Rust Scrub

Rust happens when oxygen comes in contact with bare iron. The two substances react and the iron surface becomes reddish, flaky and fragile. Thin iron objects can be completely destroyed during a short period of time. Thicker iron surfaces can be cleaned and maintained for many years. If you want to clean the rust from old utensils and kitchen pots, here is a homemade lemon scrub.

Ingredients:

¼ cup of freshly squeezed lemon juice
½ cup of thick salt

Directions:

Mix the lemon juice and the salt in a small bowl. Use the paste to scrub the rust from the iron surfaces. Leave the mixture on the iron for 5 minutes, rinse with warm water and wipe completely dry.

Conclusion

I very much hope that you found some useful things in this book. You see, the very purpose of this work was to help you see at least one small piece of the whole new way of thinking about natural products and their uses, in fields where the artificial, chemical and conventional is placed as more natural than natural itself.

Science's contribution to health, beauty and cleanliness is undisputable. But do we really need its products so much for all the minor flaws in our appearance, all the easily cured coughs and such simple things like cleaning the fridge? Maybe all these complex ingredients do more harm than good when trying to help with the little things?

As you already saw, one simple fruit can help you in not one, not ten, but in fifty ways! And don't forget that the recipes and tips you read here are only a compilation of my top 50 uses of lemon.

One last thing…

I would be delighted to hear about your experience with the lemon recipes you found useful and will be happy to discuss all of them, as well as your own recipes and tips, further with you! So do not hesitate to leave feedback. It is precious for me and always welcome! You can post your review here: http://www.amazon.com/gp/product/B019BT7WX8

As a writer, I love to hear what the readers think about my works. How do you find the book? Were there typos? Spelling errors? Or grammar issues? Let me know! If you already have written a review for this book, then send me an e-mail at nightingalelorraine@gmail.com, together with the link to the review, so that you can receive another freebie: *100+ Juice and Smoothie Recipes That Will Boost Your Energy and Cleanse Your Body!* Your review would really help me write better books in the future.

Thanks so much!